TEN EASY STEPS TO REDUCE YOUR CHOLESTEROL, BURN FAT, BALANCED DIET AND REGULAR EXERCISE IN 30 DAYS WITHOUT PRESCRIPTION DRUGS

BY

LUCIA DIAZ MATEO

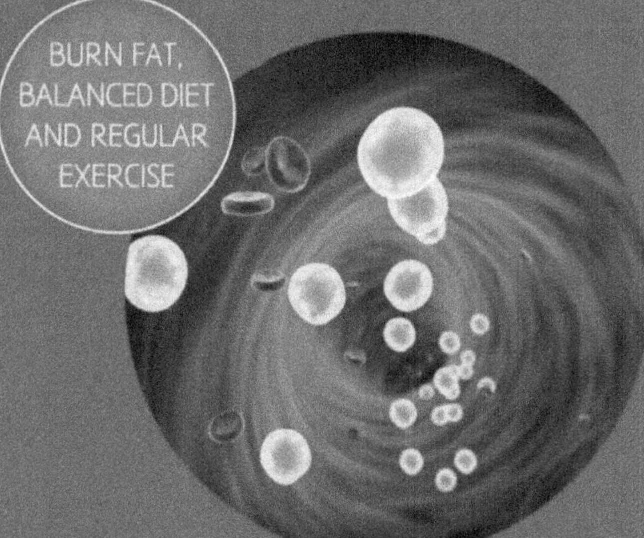

TEN EASY STEPS TO REDUCE YOUR CHOLESTEROL
BURN FAT, BALANCED DIET AND REGULAR EXERCISE
IN 30 DAYS WITHOUT PRESCRIPTION DRUGS
LUCIA DIAZ MATEO

CONTENTS

Welcome

In a world where hectic lifestyles and sedentary habits often take precedence, maintaining optimal health has become a paramount concern. The contemporary pace of life, coupled with the ubiquity of processed foods, has given rise to health challenges, with elevated cholesterol levels and excess fat deposition at the forefront. However, the journey to a healthier you doesn't have to be arduous or reliant on prescription drugs. This guide presents a transformative plan – a 30-day roadmap to reduce cholesterol, burn fat, embrace a balanced diet, and incorporate regular exercise into your daily routine, all without the need for pharmaceutical interventions.

As we delve into these ten easy steps, it's crucial to recognize that health is a holistic pursuit, encompassing not only what we eat but also how we move our bodies. The key lies in adopting sustainable lifestyle changes that contribute to overall well-being. By following this comprehensive plan, you'll discover that achieving and maintaining a healthy cholesterol level and shedding excess fat need not be a daunting task.

The approach outlined here emphasizes the power of simple, yet effective, strategies. From making mindful choices in your diet to incorporating manageable exercise routines, each step is designed to be seamlessly integrated into your existing lifestyle. Gone are the days of extreme diets and exhausting workout regimens; instead, this guide promotes a balanced and realistic approach to wellness.

Throughout the next 30 days, we will navigate the intricacies of nutrition, explore the benefits of specific foods, and unveil exercises that cater to diverse fitness levels. By the end of this transformative journey, you'll not only witness a positive shift in your cholesterol levels and fat metabolism but also experience an enhanced sense of vitality and well-rounded health.

Embark on this empowering expedition with us, as we unveil the secrets to a healthier, fitter you – all within the grasp of your daily routine and without the reliance on prescription drugs. Get ready to embrace positive change and witness the remarkable impact it can have on your life in just 30 days.

Chapter 1: Understanding Cholesterol

Cholesterol, a fatty substance found in every cell of our body, plays a crucial role in various physiological functions. While our body naturally produces cholesterol, the levels can be influenced by lifestyle factors and dietary choices. Understanding the nuances of cholesterol is the first step towards managing and reducing it effectively.

Cholesterol is classified into two main types: low-density lipoprotein (LDL) and high-density lipoprotein (HDL). LDL cholesterol, often referred to as "bad" cholesterol, can build up in the walls of arteries, leading to plaque formation and potential blockages. On the other hand, HDL cholesterol, or "good" cholesterol, helps remove LDL from the bloodstream, reducing the risk of heart disease.

Maintaining a healthy cholesterol level is vital for cardiovascular health. Elevated levels of LDL cholesterol can contribute to atherosclerosis, a condition where arteries become narrow due to the buildup of plaque. This restricts blood flow, increasing the risk of heart attacks and strokes.

Several factors can contribute to high cholesterol levels, including genetics, age, and gender. However, lifestyle choices such as diet, exercise, and smoking play a significant role in cholesterol management. Unhealthy eating habits, rich in saturated and trans fats, can elevate LDL cholesterol, while a diet high in fiber and omega-3 fatty acids can help lower it.

Understanding cholesterol numbers is essential. Total cholesterol, LDL cholesterol, HDL cholesterol, and triglycerides are the key components measured in a lipid profile. A desirable total cholesterol level is generally below 200 mg/dL, with LDL cholesterol ideally below 100 mg/dL. HDL cholesterol levels above 60 mg/dL are considered protective against heart disease.

To embark on the journey of managing cholesterol effectively, it's crucial to get regular cholesterol screenings. This provides a baseline understanding of your cholesterol levels and helps track any changes over time. Many individuals might not experience any symptoms of high cholesterol, underscoring the importance of routine check-ups.

Moreover, understanding the risk factors associated with high cholesterol is paramount. Age, family history, and pre-existing conditions such as diabetes can increase susceptibility. Awareness of these factors empowers individuals to make informed decisions about their lifestyle and dietary choices.

As you delve into the intricacies of cholesterol management, it's important to recognize that not all cholesterol is detrimental. HDL cholesterol serves a protective function by transporting excess cholesterol to the liver for removal. Thus, the focus should be on achieving a balance between LDL and HDL cholesterol, rather than aiming for extremely low total cholesterol levels.

Chapter 2: Assessing Your Current Lifestyle

Assessing your current lifestyle is a crucial first step in embarking on a journey to reduce cholesterol, burn fat, and achieve a balanced, healthy life. Our habits, both dietary and physical, play a significant role in determining our overall well-being. This aims to guide you through a comprehensive self-assessment, helping you identify areas that need improvement and setting the foundation for positive changes.

Understanding Your Current Habits

Start by taking a close look at your daily routine. What do you typically eat? How much physical activity do you engage in? Are there specific stressors in your life that might contribute to unhealthy habits? By understanding your current lifestyle, you can pinpoint areas that may be contributing to high cholesterol and excess body fat.

Dietary Analysis

Create a food diary for at least a week, documenting everything you eat and drink. Pay attention to portion sizes, meal timings, and the nutritional content of your food. Identify patterns, such as excessive consumption of saturated fats, trans fats, and refined sugars. This analysis can reveal dietary habits that may be impacting your cholesterol levels.

Physical Activity Assessment

Evaluate your current exercise routine, if any. How often do you engage in physical activity? What types of exercises do you enjoy, and how intense are they? Understanding your baseline activity level helps in designing a realistic and effective workout plan for the next 30 days.

Stress and Sleep Evaluation

Stress and inadequate sleep can contribute to elevated cholesterol levels. Assess your stress levels by identifying sources of stress in your life. Additionally, analyze your sleep patterns—how many hours of quality sleep do you get each night? Poor sleep can affect metabolism and exacerbate weight and cholesterol issues.

Identifying Risk Factors

Beyond diet and exercise, other lifestyle factors can influence cholesterol and fat levels. Evaluate the following risk factors:

Smoking and Alcohol Consumption

If you smoke or consume alcohol regularly, these habits can impact your cardiovascular health. Consider strategies for reducing or eliminating these habits during the next 30 days.

Genetics and Family History

Understanding your family's medical history, especially regarding heart disease and cholesterol issues, provides insights into your own risk factors. If there's a family predisposition, taking proactive measures becomes even more crucial.

Body Mass Index (BMI) and Waist Circumference

Calculate your BMI and measure your waist circumference. Excess body weight, especially around the abdomen, is often associated with higher cholesterol levels and increased cardiovascular risk.

Setting Realistic Goals

Based on your assessment, establish achievable short-term goals for the next 30 days. These goals should be specific, measurable, and tailored to your individual lifestyle. For example:

- Dietary Goals: Reduce saturated fat intake, increase fiber consumption, and limit added sugars.

- Exercise Goals: Aim for at least 150 minutes of moderate-intensity aerobic exercise per week, along with strength training exercises.

- Stress Reduction Goals: Incorporate stress-relief activities, such as meditation or yoga, into your daily routine.

- Sleep Goals: Prioritize sleep by creating a consistent sleep schedule and creating a calming bedtime routine.

Creating an Action Plan

With a clear understanding of your current lifestyle, risk factors, and realistic goals, it's time to develop a personalized action plan. This plan should outline specific steps you will take each day to achieve your objectives. Consider involving a healthcare professional or a nutritionist to ensure your plan aligns with your health needs and goals.

Chapter 3: Planning a Balanced Diet

A balanced diet plays a pivotal role in managing cholesterol levels and promoting overall health. the components of a well-rounded diet that supports your cardiovascular well-being. By making thoughtful choices in your daily nutrition, you can actively contribute to lowering cholesterol, burning fat, and fostering a healthier lifestyle.

Understanding Nutrient Categories

A balanced diet encompasses a variety of essential nutrients: carbohydrates, proteins, fats, vitamins, and minerals. Striking the right balance among these categories is key to maintaining optimal health. Let's explore how each nutrient contributes to your well-being.

1. Carbohydrates:
   Carbohydrates are your body's primary energy source. Opt for complex carbohydrates found in whole grains, fruits, and vegetables. These provide sustained energy, helping to regulate blood sugar levels and prevent overeating.

2. Proteins:
   Proteins are crucial for muscle repair and overall body function. Include lean protein sources such as poultry, fish,

legumes, and tofu. These options are lower in saturated fats, promoting heart health.

3. Fats:

While fats have a bad reputation, not all fats are harmful. Focus on unsaturated fats found in avocados, nuts, seeds, and olive oil. Limit saturated and trans fats, often present in processed foods, fried items, and certain animal products.

4. Vitamins and Minerals:

A diverse diet ensures you receive a spectrum of essential vitamins and minerals. These micronutrients support various bodily functions, including immune health, bone strength, and antioxidant defense.

Cholesterol-Friendly Foods

Incorporating specific foods known for their cholesterol-lowering properties is a smart strategy. Consider these options as staples in your balanced diet:

1. Oats and Barley:

Rich in soluble fiber, oats and barley help lower LDL (bad) cholesterol levels. They can be part of a wholesome breakfast or added to soups and stews.

2. Fruits and Vegetables:

Packed with vitamins, minerals, and antioxidants, fruits and vegetables contribute to heart health. Berries, citrus fruits, leafy greens, and cruciferous vegetables are particularly beneficial.

3. Fatty Fish:
Omega-3 fatty acids, found in fatty fish like salmon and mackerel, play a vital role in reducing triglycerides and supporting heart function. Aim for at least two servings per week.

4. Nuts and Seeds:
Almonds, walnuts, flaxseeds, and chia seeds are excellent sources of healthy fats, fiber, and plant-based proteins. These can be sprinkled on salads, yogurt, or enjoyed as snacks.

5. Legumes:
Beans, lentils, and chickpeas are rich in soluble fiber and plant-based proteins, contributing to lower cholesterol levels and improved blood sugar control.

Portion Control and Moderation

While choosing nutrient-dense foods is crucial, so is controlling portion sizes. Overeating, even with healthy foods, can lead to weight gain and an imbalance in nutrient intake. Use smaller plates, listen to your body's hunger cues, and savor each bite mindfully.

Meal Planning for Success

Effective meal planning is at the core of a balanced diet. Consider the following tips when structuring your meals:

1. Frequent, Small Meals:
    Eating smaller, well-balanced meals throughout the day can help stabilize blood sugar levels and prevent overeating.

2. Colorful Plate:
    Aim for a variety of colors on your plate, indicating a diverse range of nutrients. This approach ensures you receive a broad spectrum of vitamins and minerals.

3. Hydration:
    Don't forget the importance of staying hydrated. Water aids digestion, supports metabolism, and helps maintain overall health.

4. Limit Processed Foods:
    Processed foods often contain unhealthy fats, excessive sodium, and added sugars. Minimize their presence in your diet and focus on whole, natural foods.

Personalizing Your Diet Plan

Every individual is unique, and dietary needs can vary. Consider consulting with a nutritionist or healthcare professional to tailor a balanced diet plan that suits your specific requirements, taking into account factors such as age, gender, activity level, and any existing health conditions.

Chapter 4: Incorporating Superfoods for Heart Health

Maintaining a heart-healthy lifestyle involves more than just cutting back on certain foods; it's equally important to include nutrient-dense superfoods that actively contribute to reducing cholesterol levels and promoting overall cardiovascular well-being.

explore a variety of superfoods known for their cholesterol-lowering and heart-protective properties, providing you with a comprehensive guide to integrating them into your daily diet.

1. Oats and Barley:
Start your day with a bowl of oatmeal or barley. These whole grains are rich in beta-glucans, a type of soluble fiber that helps lower LDL (low-density lipoprotein) cholesterol levels. The soluble fiber in oats and barley forms a gel-like substance in the digestive tract, preventing the absorption of cholesterol into the bloodstream.

2. Fatty Fish:
Include fatty fish like salmon, mackerel, and trout in your diet at least twice a week. These fish are abundant in omega-3 fatty acids, which have been shown to reduce triglycerides, lower blood pressure, and decrease the risk of blood clot formation. Omega-3 fatty acids also contribute to

maintaining a healthy balance of HDL (high-density lipoprotein) and LDL cholesterol.

3. Nuts and Seeds:
Snack on a handful of nuts, such as almonds, walnuts, or pistachios, to add heart-healthy monounsaturated and polyunsaturated fats to your diet. These fats can help lower LDL cholesterol levels. Additionally, nuts and seeds are excellent sources of plant sterols, which can further contribute to reducing cholesterol absorption in the body.

4. Avocados:
Incorporate avocados into your meals for a dose of monounsaturated fats, potassium, and fiber. Avocados can help lower LDL cholesterol and raise HDL cholesterol levels. They are versatile and can be added to salads, sandwiches, or enjoyed as a tasty spread.

5. Berries:
Berries, such as strawberries, blueberries, and raspberries, are packed with antioxidants, fiber, and vitamins. These components work together to improve heart health by reducing inflammation, lowering blood pressure, and enhancing overall cardiovascular function.

6. Garlic:
Add garlic to your dishes for both flavor and health benefits. Garlic contains allicin, a compound known for its

anti-inflammatory and antioxidant properties. It can help lower cholesterol levels and reduce blood pressure, contributing to a healthier cardiovascular system.

7. Olive Oil:

Switch to extra virgin olive oil as your primary cooking oil. Rich in monounsaturated fats and antioxidants, olive oil has been associated with lower levels of LDL cholesterol. Use it in salad dressings, sautéing, or drizzle it over vegetables for a heart-healthy boost.

8. Leafy Greens:

Include dark leafy greens like spinach, kale, and Swiss chard in your meals. These vegetables are high in fiber, vitamins, and minerals, promoting heart health. They also contain antioxidants that combat oxidative stress and inflammation.

9. Beans and Legumes:

Beans, lentils, and other legumes are excellent sources of soluble fiber, which helps lower cholesterol levels. They are also low in saturated fats and provide essential nutrients like potassium and magnesium, beneficial for maintaining cardiovascular health.

10. Green Tea:

Swap sugary beverages with green tea, a rich source of antioxidants called catechins. Regular consumption of green tea has been linked to lower LDL cholesterol levels and improved arterial function. Aim for at least one or two cups a day for optimal benefits.

11. Dark Chocolate:
Indulge in dark chocolate with at least 70% cocoa content. Dark chocolate contains flavonoids, which have been associated with improved heart health. Consumed in moderation, dark chocolate may contribute to lower blood pressure and improved blood vessel function.

12. Tomatoes:
Tomatoes are rich in lycopene, an antioxidant that gives them their vibrant red color. Lycopene has been linked to lower LDL cholesterol levels and a reduced risk of heart disease. Enjoy tomatoes in salads, sauces, or as a snack for added cardiovascular benefits.

Incorporating these superfoods into your diet can significantly contribute to reducing cholesterol levels and improving overall heart health. Remember to maintain variety in your meals to ensure you receive a broad spectrum of nutrients essential for optimal cardiovascular function. As always, consult with a healthcare professional or a nutritionist before making significant dietary changes, especially if you have existing health conditions or are taking medication.

Chapter 5: Crafting Effective Meal Plans for Cholesterol Management

Maintaining a balanced and heart-healthy diet is paramount when aiming to reduce cholesterol levels and promote overall well-being. the intricacies of crafting effective meal plans that prioritize nutrient-rich foods while minimizing cholesterol-raising elements.

The Foundation of a Heart-Healthy Diet

Your meal plan's foundation should consist of whole, unprocessed foods. These include fruits, vegetables, whole grains, lean proteins, and healthy fats. These foods provide essential nutrients, fiber, and antioxidants that support cardiovascular health.

1. Fruits and Vegetables

Incorporate a colorful array of fruits and vegetables into your meals. These foods are rich in vitamins, minerals, and antioxidants that combat inflammation and oxidative stress. Aim for at least 5 servings a day, emphasizing leafy greens, berries, citrus fruits, and cruciferous vegetables.

2. Whole Grains

Choose whole grains over refined grains to boost fiber intake. Oats, quinoa, brown rice, and whole wheat are excellent choices. Fiber helps lower cholesterol levels by reducing the absorption of dietary cholesterol and improving overall heart health.

3. Lean Proteins

Include lean protein sources in your meals, such as poultry, fish, legumes, and tofu. These options are lower in saturated fats, which can contribute to elevated cholesterol levels. Fatty fish like salmon and trout also provide omega-3 fatty acids, known for their heart-protective properties.

4. Healthy Fats

Opt for heart-healthy fats like those found in avocados, nuts, seeds, and olive oil. These fats help raise HDL (good) cholesterol while lowering LDL (bad) cholesterol. However, moderation is key, as fats are calorie-dense.

Meal Planning Strategies

1. Portion Control

Managing portion sizes is crucial for weight control and cholesterol management. Use smaller plates, and be mindful of portion sizes to avoid overeating. This simple strategy can make a significant difference in calorie intake.

2. Regular Meal Timing

Establishing regular meal times helps regulate blood sugar levels and prevents excessive snacking. Aim for three balanced meals and consider incorporating healthy snacks if needed. Consistency in meal timing supports overall metabolic health.

3. Limiting Processed Foods

Processed foods often contain trans fats and high levels of sodium, which can negatively impact cholesterol levels and cardiovascular health. Minimize your intake of packaged snacks, fast food, and sugary beverages.

Sample Heart-Healthy Meal Plan

Breakfast:
- Oatmeal with sliced strawberries and almonds
- Greek yogurt with a drizzle of honey
- Green tea or black coffee

Lunch:
- Grilled chicken or tofu salad with mixed greens, cherry tomatoes, and quinoa

- Olive oil and balsamic vinegar dressing
- A small apple or pear

Snack:
- Carrot sticks with hummus
- A handful of walnuts or almonds

Dinner:
- Baked salmon or lentil stew
- Steamed broccoli and quinoa
- Mixed berry dessert with a dollop of Greek yogurt

Note: Adapt this plan based on your individual dietary preferences, caloric needs, and any specific health considerations.

Consulting a Nutritionist

While these guidelines offer a general framework, it's advisable to consult with a registered dietitian or nutritionist for a personalized approach. They can assess your specific needs, preferences, and potential dietary restrictions, ensuring that your meal plan aligns with your health goals.

Chapter 6: Smart Snacking Choices for Cholesterol Management

Snacking can be a stumbling block or a stepping stone on your journey to lower cholesterol and overall well-being. Making mindful choices during snack time is crucial in maintaining a balanced diet and achieving your health goals.

the importance of smart snacking, identify wholesome options, and offer tips on incorporating these choices into your daily routine.

Understanding Smart Snacking

Snacking, when done right, can provide essential nutrients, regulate blood sugar levels, and prevent overeating during main meals. Smart snacking involves choosing foods that contribute to your overall health, rather than opting for sugary, processed, or high-saturated-fat snacks that may raise cholesterol levels.

Ideal Components of Smart Snacks

1. Fiber-Rich Foods:
    Incorporate snacks high in soluble fiber, such as fruits, vegetables, and whole grains. Soluble fiber helps lower LDL

cholesterol levels by binding to cholesterol molecules and aiding in their elimination from the body.

2. Healthy Fats:
   Opt for snacks containing unsaturated fats, like those found in nuts, seeds, and avocados. These fats can help raise HDL (good) cholesterol and lower LDL (bad) cholesterol.

3. Protein Sources:
   Including protein in your snacks can promote satiety and prevent excessive calorie intake. Consider options like Greek yogurt, lean meats, or legumes.

4. Antioxidant-Rich Choices:
   Snacks loaded with antioxidants, such as berries, dark chocolate, and green tea, can combat oxidative stress and inflammation, contributing to heart health.

5. Portion Control:
   Be mindful of portion sizes to avoid overconsumption. Pre-portion snacks or choose snacks that come in convenient single servings to prevent mindless eating.

Healthy Snack Ideas

1. Fresh Fruit with Nut Butter:

Pairing apple slices or banana with almond or peanut butter provides a satisfying mix of fiber, vitamins, and healthy fats.

2. Vegetable Sticks with Hummus:
Crunchy veggies like carrots, cucumber, and bell peppers combined with hummus offer a nutrient-packed, low-calorie snack.

3. Greek Yogurt Parfait:
Layering Greek yogurt with berries and a sprinkle of nuts creates a tasty, protein-rich snack that supports heart health.

4. Oatmeal Cookies:
Prepare homemade oatmeal cookies using whole-grain oats, nuts, and dried fruits for a delicious and heart-friendly treat.

5. Trail Mix:
Create a customized trail mix with a mix of nuts, seeds, and dried fruits. This snack is portable, convenient, and provides a good balance of nutrients.

Tips for Incorporating Smart Snacking into Your Routine

1. Plan Ahead:

Preparing snacks in advance helps you make mindful choices and prevents reaching for less healthy options when hunger strikes.

2. Hydration:

Often, our bodies confuse thirst with hunger. Stay adequately hydrated throughout the day to reduce the likelihood of unnecessary snacking.

3. Read Labels:

Be vigilant about reading nutritional labels to understand the ingredients and make informed choices. Look for snacks low in added sugars and saturated fats.

4. Mindful Eating:

Take time to savor your snacks, appreciating the flavors and textures. This practice helps you stay connected with your body's hunger and fullness cues.

5. Variety is Key:

Keep your snacking routine interesting by rotating through different options. This not only provides a diverse range of nutrients but also prevents boredom.

Chapter 7: The Role of Exercise in Cholesterol Management

Physical activity is a cornerstone of a healthy lifestyle, especially when it comes to managing cholesterol levels. Regular exercise not only contributes to burning fat but also plays a crucial role in raising HDL (high-density lipoprotein) cholesterol, the "good" cholesterol, while lowering LDL (low-density lipoprotein) cholesterol, the "bad" cholesterol. In this chapter, we'll delve into the various ways exercise impacts cholesterol and explore effective workout routines for achieving optimal results.

Understanding Cholesterol and Exercise:

Cholesterol is a fatty substance that is essential for building cells and producing certain hormones. However, an imbalance in cholesterol levels, particularly elevated LDL cholesterol, can lead to atherosclerosis, a condition where cholesterol deposits build up on artery walls, increasing the risk of heart disease.

Exercise influences cholesterol levels through several mechanisms. Firstly, it promotes weight loss and the reduction of excess body fat. Since cholesterol is stored in fat cells, shedding those extra pounds can lead to a decrease in overall cholesterol levels.

Secondly, physical activity increases the production of HDL cholesterol. HDL acts as a scavenger, collecting excess cholesterol from the blood vessels and transporting it to the liver for excretion. This process helps prevent cholesterol buildup in the arteries.

Choosing the Right Exercise:

Not all exercises are created equal when it comes to managing cholesterol. Aerobic exercises, also known as cardiovascular or endurance exercises, are particularly effective. These include activities like brisk walking, jogging, cycling, swimming, and dancing. Aim for at least 150 minutes of moderate-intensity aerobic exercise per week, or 75 minutes of vigorous-intensity exercise, spread throughout the week.

Strength training or resistance exercises are also beneficial. Building muscle mass can improve your body's ability to metabolize fats and sugars, which, in turn, can positively impact cholesterol levels. Incorporate strength training activities, such as weightlifting or bodyweight exercises, at least two days a week.

Creating a Balanced Workout Routine:

To maximize the cholesterol-lowering benefits of exercise, it's essential to incorporate a variety of activities into your routine. This not only keeps things interesting but also engages different muscle groups and energy systems. Consider a weekly schedule that includes a mix of aerobic exercises, strength training, and flexibility exercises like yoga or Pilates.

For cardiovascular health, aim for activities that elevate your heart rate and make you breathe harder. This could be a brisk walk, a jog, or a cycling session. Start with moderate-intensity workouts and gradually increase the intensity as your fitness level improves.

When it comes to strength training, focus on major muscle groups such as legs, back, chest, and core. Include exercises like squats, lunges, push-ups, and planks. Using a variety of equipment, such as dumbbells, resistance bands, or your body weight, can add diversity to your routine.

Tips for Effective Exercise:

1. Consistency is Key: Establish a regular exercise routine and stick to it. Consistency is crucial for long-term benefits.

2. Start Slow: If you're new to exercise or haven't been active for a while, start with low-intensity activities and gradually progress. This reduces the risk of injury and makes the routine more sustainable.

3. Mix It Up: Keep your workouts interesting by incorporating different activities. This not only prevents boredom but also ensures that you engage various muscle groups.

4. Set Realistic Goals: Define achievable fitness goals and track your progress. Celebrate small victories along the way to stay motivated.

5. Listen to Your Body: Pay attention to how your body responds to exercise. If you experience pain or discomfort, modify your routine or consult a fitness professional.

6. Stay Hydrated: Proper hydration is essential for overall health and can enhance the effectiveness of your workouts.

7. Include Rest Days: Give your body time to recover. Rest days are crucial for preventing burnout and reducing the risk of overuse injuries.

Combining Exercise with a Healthy Diet:

While exercise is a powerful tool for managing cholesterol, its benefits are amplified when combined with a healthy diet. A balanced diet rich in fruits, vegetables, whole grains, and lean proteins complements the positive effects of regular physical activity. Together, they create a synergistic approach to cholesterol management.

Chapter 8: Creating a Sustainable Workout Routine

Maintaining a regular exercise routine is crucial for managing cholesterol levels and promoting overall cardiovascular health. the specifics of crafting a sustainable workout plan that not only burns fat but also fits seamlessly into your daily life.

The Importance of Exercise

Exercise has multifaceted benefits for your health, and when it comes to cholesterol management, it plays a pivotal role. Regular physical activity helps raise high-density lipoprotein (HDL) cholesterol, often referred to as the "good" cholesterol, which works to carry cholesterol away from the arteries and back to the liver for processing or excretion.

Additionally, exercise aids in weight management. Shedding excess weight contributes to lower levels of low-density lipoprotein (LDL) cholesterol, the "bad" cholesterol responsible for building up in the arteries. This reduction in LDL cholesterol diminishes the risk of atherosclerosis, a condition characterized by the hardening and narrowing of arteries due to cholesterol deposits.

Types of Exercise

A well-rounded workout routine should include both aerobic exercises and strength training. Aerobic exercises, such as walking, jogging, swimming, or cycling, elevate your heart rate and contribute to burning calories and improving cardiovascular health. Aim for at least 150 minutes of moderate-intensity aerobic exercise per week or 75 minutes of vigorous-intensity exercise.

Strength training, on the other hand, helps build muscle mass, which can enhance your body's ability to burn calories even when at rest. Engage in strength training activities like weightlifting or bodyweight exercises at least twice a week, targeting major muscle groups.

Crafting Your Routine

1. Start Slow:
   If you're new to exercise or haven't been active for a while, it's essential to start slowly. Gradually increase the intensity and duration of your workouts to prevent injuries and make the process more sustainable.

2. Choose Activities You Enjoy:
   The key to maintaining a long-term exercise routine is finding activities you genuinely enjoy. Whether it's dancing,

hiking, or playing a sport, incorporating activities you love increases the likelihood of sticking to your routine.

3. Mix It Up:

Variety is not only the spice of life but also the essence of a sustainable workout routine. Keep things interesting by incorporating different activities throughout the week. This not only prevents boredom but also ensures that you engage various muscle groups.

4. Set Realistic Goals:

Establish achievable short-term and long-term fitness goals. Whether it's running a certain distance, lifting a specific weight, or completing a set number of push-ups, setting realistic goals provides motivation and a sense of accomplishment.

5. Schedule Regular Workouts:

Consistency is key. Schedule your workouts just like any other appointment. This not only helps form a habit but also ensures that exercise becomes an integral part of your routine.

6. Include Both Cardio and Strength Training:

Balance is crucial. Incorporate a mix of aerobic exercises and strength training in your routine to address different aspects of cardiovascular health and overall fitness.

Sample Weekly Workout Plan

Monday:
- 30 minutes of brisk walking or jogging
- Bodyweight exercises (push-ups, squats, lunges) - 20 minutes

Tuesday:
- Swimming or cycling - 30 minutes
- Yoga or stretching - 15 minutes

Wednesday:
- Strength training (weightlifting or resistance training) - 30 minutes
- 15 minutes of high-intensity interval training (HIIT)

Thursday:
- Rest day or light activity (such as walking or gentle yoga)

Friday:
- 45 minutes of moderate-intensity cardio (running, elliptical, or cycling)
- Core exercises (planks, crunches) - 15 minutes

Saturday:
- Hiking or outdoor activity - 1 hour
- Relaxing activities like meditation or gentle stretching - 15 minutes

Sunday:
- Rest day or light activity

Listening to Your Body

While having a structured workout plan is essential, it's equally important to listen to your body. If you feel fatigued or experience pain, it's crucial to rest and allow your body to recover. Overtraining can lead to burnout and may have adverse effects on your overall health.

Chapter 9: Stress Management Techniques

In the hustle and bustle of our daily lives, stress has become an omnipresent companion. Unfortunately, chronic stress can significantly impact our health, including cholesterol levels. The effective stress management techniques to help you maintain a balanced and heart-healthy lifestyle.

Understanding the Stress-Cholesterol Connection:

Stress triggers the release of hormones like cortisol, which can lead to increased levels of cholesterol in the bloodstream. Additionally, stress may contribute to unhealthy coping mechanisms such as overeating or indulging in comfort foods, which can further impact cholesterol levels. Recognizing this connection is the first step towards implementing strategies to manage stress effectively.

Mindfulness Meditation:

One powerful technique for stress reduction is mindfulness meditation. This practice involves focusing your attention on the present moment without judgment. Regular mindfulness meditation has been shown to lower stress levels, improve emotional well-being, and even positively impact cholesterol profiles. Consider incorporating short meditation sessions into your daily routine to experience these benefits.

Deep Breathing Exercises:

Deep breathing exercises are a simple yet effective way to activate the body's relaxation response. Practice diaphragmatic breathing by inhaling deeply through your nose, allowing your abdomen to expand, and exhaling slowly through your mouth. This technique can be done anywhere, making it a convenient tool for managing stress in various situations.

Regular Physical Activity:

Exercise is not only crucial for maintaining overall health but also plays a vital role in stress management. Physical activity prompts the release of endorphins, the body's natural mood lifters. Aim for at least 30 minutes of moderate-intensity exercise most days of the week. Whether it's brisk walking, jogging, cycling, or yoga, find activities you enjoy to make exercise a sustainable part of your routine.

Social Support:

Sharing your feelings and experiences with friends, family, or a support group can provide emotional relief and foster a sense of connection. Strong social networks act as a buffer against stress, and the support of loved ones can make challenging situations more manageable. Prioritize spending quality time with those who uplift and support you.

Time Management Strategies:

Feeling overwhelmed by a hectic schedule can contribute to chronic stress. Implementing effective time management strategies can help create a sense of control and reduce stress levels. Prioritize tasks, break them into smaller, manageable steps, and delegate when possible. This can prevent the accumulation of stressors and provide a more balanced approach to daily responsibilities.

Cognitive Behavioral Therapy (CBT):

For those dealing with chronic stress or anxiety, cognitive-behavioral therapy can be a valuable tool. CBT helps individuals identify and change negative thought patterns and behaviors that contribute to stress. Working with a trained therapist can provide personalized strategies to cope with stress and improve overall mental well-being.

Hobbies and Leisure Activities:

Engaging in hobbies and activities you enjoy can be a powerful antidote to stress. Whether it's reading, gardening, painting, or playing a musical instrument, dedicating time to activities that bring joy and relaxation can positively impact your mood and help alleviate stress.

Adequate Sleep:

Quality sleep is crucial for overall health and stress management. Lack of sleep can contribute to heightened stress levels and negatively impact cholesterol levels. Establish a consistent sleep routine, create a comfortable sleep environment, and aim for 7-9 hours of sleep per night to support both your mental and cardiovascular health.

Balanced Nutrition for Stress Resilience:

Just as your diet plays a role in managing cholesterol, it also influences your response to stress. Ensure your diet includes nutrient-dense foods that support brain health and provide a steady release of energy. Foods rich in omega-3 fatty acids, antioxidants, and complex carbohydrates can contribute to stress resilience.

Chapter 10: Quality Sleep for Better Health

Sleep is a fundamental aspect of overall well-being, playing a crucial role in maintaining physical, mental, and emotional health. When it comes to managing cholesterol levels and promoting heart health, the significance of quality sleep cannot be overstated. In this chapter, we will explore the intricate relationship between sleep and cholesterol, understand how sleep impacts our body, and discuss practical tips to ensure a restful night's sleep.

Understanding the Connection: Sleep and Cholesterol

Numerous studies have established a clear link between insufficient sleep and unfavorable changes in cholesterol levels. Sleep deprivation or poor-quality sleep can lead to an increase in low-density lipoprotein (LDL) cholesterol, commonly known as "bad" cholesterol. Additionally, it may result in lower levels of high-density lipoprotein (HDL) cholesterol, often referred to as "good" cholesterol.

The mechanism behind this connection involves disruptions in the body's internal biological clock, which regulates various metabolic processes, including cholesterol metabolism. When sleep is compromised, the body's ability to process and regulate cholesterol is hindered, contributing to an imbalance in cholesterol levels.

Impact of Sleep on Metabolism and Weight Management

Beyond its direct influence on cholesterol, sleep also plays a pivotal role in metabolic processes and weight management. Sleep deprivation can disrupt the balance of hormones that regulate hunger and satiety, leading to increased cravings for unhealthy, high-calorie foods. Over time, this can contribute to weight gain and obesity, both of which are risk factors for elevated cholesterol levels.

Furthermore, inadequate sleep can impair insulin sensitivity, promoting insulin resistance. This, in turn, may contribute to metabolic syndrome—a cluster of conditions that includes high blood pressure, high blood sugar, excess body fat around the waist, and abnormal cholesterol levels.

Practical Strategies for Improving Sleep Quality

1. Establish a Consistent Sleep Schedule:
   Set a regular sleep-wake cycle by going to bed and waking up at the same time every day, even on weekends. This helps regulate your body's internal clock.

2. Create a Relaxing Bedtime Routine:
      Develop pre-sleep rituals such as reading a book, practicing relaxation techniques, or taking a warm bath. These activities signal to your body that it's time to wind down.

3. Optimize Sleep Environment:
   Ensure your bedroom is conducive to sleep by keeping it cool, dark, and quiet. Invest in a comfortable mattress and pillows to enhance overall comfort.

4. Limit Exposure to Screens Before Bed:
   The blue light emitted by electronic devices can interfere with the production of the sleep hormone melatonin. Aim to reduce screen time at least an hour before bedtime.

5. Watch Your Diet:
   Avoid heavy meals, caffeine, and nicotine close to bedtime. Opt for a light snack if you're hungry before sleep, and stay hydrated throughout the day.

6. Regular Exercise:
   Engage in regular physical activity, but try to complete your workout at least a few hours before bedtime. Exercise promotes better sleep, but intense activity too close to bedtime may have the opposite effect.

7. Manage Stress:
   Incorporate stress-reducing techniques such as meditation, deep breathing exercises, or yoga into your daily routine. Managing stress can significantly improve sleep quality.

8. Limit Naps:

While short naps can be rejuvenating, avoid napping for extended periods during the day, as it may interfere with nighttime sleep.

Monitoring Progress and Seeking Professional Guidance

As you implement these strategies, it's essential to monitor your sleep patterns and make adjustments as needed. Keep a sleep diary to track the duration and quality of your sleep, as well as any factors that may be affecting it. If sleep problems persist despite your efforts, it may be prudent to consult with a healthcare professional or a sleep specialist for further evaluation.

Author Bio

Lucia Diaz Mateo, a distinguished endocrinologist specializing in gestational diabetes and women's health, is the accomplished author behind this comprehensive guide. Holding a Doctorate in Medicine from a renowned institution, Lucia Diaz Mateo,
 has dedicated her career to advancing the understanding and management of healthy living.

With a passion for patient-centric care, Lucia Diaz Mateo, combines her extensive clinical experience with a commitment to educating and empowering women. Her research contributions have been widely recognized in leading medical journals, solidifying her position as a respected authority in the field.